Thinkwich

i

Thinkwich

Supporting the Psychological Well-Being of the Elderly.

Triggering Thoughts of the Past, Alongside the Thinking Still Needed For Today.

A.C French.

Published by Lulu

<u>Copyright Information</u>

Preface

The cognitive decline associated with old age is part of why this book was written. The other driving force behind the conception and publication of *Thinkwich* was the COVID-19 pandemic; specifically, how the pandemic prevented me, and others in our family from regularly travelling to see our mother, who lives alone in her retirement community in Spain. This creating a heightened sense of concern for us, bearing in mind our mother is in her eighty-ninth year.

She had also been very candid, regarding the fact that she was forgetting things more often than before, this sometimes including special dates, or whether she had done certain tasks for instance.

As a result of the lock downs and travel restrictions the frequency of video calls between us increased. After a time I noticed that the general everyday questions I was asking, whilst eliciting a response, were generally failing to lift her spirits. This was exacerbated by the increased isolation our mother was enduring; isolation that was not limited to family, as on various occasions, she was also prevented from seeing her friends.

Later, during another video call, I was updating her on news regarding a grandson and some recently enjoyed soccer success, when the conversation took a turn back to her grandfather and how he had been a very well-known footballer in his day.

I remember half-noticing her increased level of engagement as she described in some detail his background, some of the team's successes, and other points of interest at the time, but I didn't think much more of it as we then continued our conversation along more general lines and said our goodbyes.

That evening, it struck me again how much more upbeat than usual my mother had sounded in the later stages of the video call. I thought back to the call and definitely sensed an increased sense of engagement, *even on the minor topics* we had closed on; **this got me thinking.**

To cut a long story short, I began to research into the nature of *remote* memory (memories made in the distant past) and also *recent* memory, so important for day-to-day life, learning, reasoning, performing tasks and overall cognitive function.

This juxtaposition of *remote* and *recent* memory became the foundation for *Thinkwich.* After considerable trial, error, and evolution, the book now hopefully represents more than just an idea conceived to help our mother and her sense of well-being.

I truly hope that in time *you* will feel that picking up a copy of *Thinkwich,* was a worthwhile decision and that it may have contributed in some way to the sense of well-being enjoyed by an elderly loved one of yours.

<u>Acknowledgements</u>

Thank you to Mrs. Pat French and friends at Ciudad Patricia retirement community in Benidorm, Spain. Without your feedback and participation, *Thinkwich* would never have been published. Many thanks also to Young Joo, John, Jane, Harley, and Alison; you each helped more than you might have realized. Thanks again for your thoughts, feedback, and ongoing support and encouragement.

Contents

Chapter	Pg.

1. About *Thinkwich*.

Thinkwich is a book of specially arranged questions a family can use to stimulate increased mental activity on the part of an elderly relative, who may be experiencing some form of age-related cognitive difficulty. This may range from frustration with increasing forgetfulness or other concerns, to more serious cognitive impairment.

The book may also be of use in cases of post-stroke recovery and *part-use* in cases of Alzheimer's disease and other forms of dementia. The term *part-use* being important in the case of dementia, as there are questions in the book that require the use of reasoning, which of course will need to be avoided.

The book, represents an inspiring way for the family and the senior concerned, to create and maintain stimulating communication and interaction experiences together. The family, can use the specially designed question lists as a resource to stimulate deeper thinking and mental activity, on the part of an aged loved one. Whether this is in a face-to-face setting, a video call, or even just a regular telephone call. or even just a regular telephone call.

Why?

Whatever the setting, the challenge is to help improve the chances that an elderly relative will retain mental acuity and a sense of well-being for as long as possible.

This is bearing in mind the effects of any cognitive decline are likely to become more with the passage of time.

Cognitive decline in the elderly can be natural and age-related, or it can be the result of more serious underlying conditions. There are many factors that can affect the extent and progression of cognitive decline; two main areas in this regard are the *level of mental activity* enjoyed by an individual, along with the *level of social interaction.*

The two variables mentioned above, were key considerations behind the creation of *Thinkwich.*

Everyday Questions

When interacting with an elderly relative, it is of course natural to ask what could be called *everyday questions,* such as who else has been in touch, what's been on TV, or about the state of the weather. However, while obviously important to the relationship, questions of this nature are unlikely to test or stimulate the senior's capacity for deeper thought. Moreover, they are also questions that are likely to be asked on a very frequent basis, after all, they are just *everyday questions.*

Monologues

There exists also the opportunity to engage in largely one-sided conversations or monologues that simply provide an update of what's been going on in one's own life.

While this is clearly informative and will no doubt be appreciated by the elderly relative, communication of this nature is unlikely to test or stimulate deeper thinking.

The Goal Is Increased Engagement

Thinkwich aims to increase the senior's engagement in the call or visit by providing thought-provoking questions for the family to ask. Questions that allow the elderly relative to open up and share details about specific events or personal experiences that occurred many years ago. These questions are then interleaved with more general questions or those related to memory and logic.

Reminiscence

Reminiscence is the thinking about or sharing of life experiences and stories about the past. In some instances, primarily involving the treatment of *Alzheimer's disease and dementia,* the act of reminiscence, can engender feelings of greater competence, confidence, well-being and also help with depression.

Despite the fact that *Thinkwich* wasn't initially conceived to help those suffering from the more severe cognitive disorders, reminiscence was still a key factor in the book's design. This is because of the positive effect reminiscence can have on *lifting the spirits* of those who engage in it.

Why *Think'wich'* ?

The book's questions stimulate remote memory and also test logic, recall and knowledge of the present or recent past. Questions have been arranged so that those requiring remote memory are sand*wiched* between those involving logic, or more recent memory, and general topics.

Rationale Behind *Thinkwich*

During our research, it became apparent that reminiscing over life events from long ago proved to be much more interesting to a senior than general questions about the *"here and now"* as it were.

The issue is of course, that the seniors, along with everyone else, are obviously living and functioning in the present. So, while reminiscence can help with recall and create a sense of well-being, there is also a need to address the mental acuity surrounding the present and more recent past; areas directly associated with living daily life.

So, we wanted to create a book that helped the senior use his or her long-term memory—*the fun bit*—alongside the more recent or short-term memory that is so *essential* for carrying out the functions of daily life.

In essence, we are using the *heightened* engagement created by the remote memory firing up to also stimulate engagement with respect to the other, more general, logic- or memory-based questions.

About The Questions

The questions are not overly country-specific, in the hope that the book can enjoy a broader appeal. We have used a mixture of US English and standard English throughout, rather than creating separate books for each.

Questions about grandchildren have not been included; this is largely because grandchildren are already likely to be a general topic of conversation. *Questions concerning partners have not been included out of respect for privacy.*

Note again: that questions in the book that require the use of reasoning must not be used in cases of dementia in any of its forms.

No Set Age Group

It is not practical to suggest a specific age group for which the book may be best suited, as each personal situation is so different. Bearing this in mind, the *family* is best placed to know whether *Thinkwich* is of interest and could potentially help *their* senior relative.

While this book is not intended for use with an elderly relative who is still *totally* mentally sharp, it may still be useful and entertaining for the senior in question to take a trip down memory lane, even if some questions may appear to be too easy.

2. Cognitive Considerations.

With the passage of time, our elderly relatives can obviously face increasingly significant challenges. Family members are likely to be aware of many of these challenges, however, there is often only so much that can be done to help; after all, old age is what it is.

There are several issues to consider when it comes to mental acuity, or mental sharpness. These include but are not limited to mild cognitive impairment (MCI), Alzheimer's or Parkinson's disease, and dementia.

Mild cognitive impairment, while not incapacitating, can still complicate life and cause stress for the senior in question. Symptoms may commonly involve losing things, forgetting appointments, or being less able to come up with words than others of a similar age.

MCI is often found to be the first stage in the progression to more serious complications. This progression can lead to more serious issues with recall, reasoning, and judgment. Coordination, motor skills, and other factors needed for social interaction and managing daily life can also be affected.

There are also potential psychological effects to consider, such as personality changes, anxiety, agitation, and depression, for instance.

Coming to terms with such a situation would almost certainly cause significant distress for the family and of course, the elderly relative in question.

There are other factors apart from age that contribute to cognitive decline, such as leading a sedentary or isolated lifestyle, high blood pressure, an insufficient amount of sleep, or a poor diet for instance. In any eventuality, it seems that the proverbial cards are generally stacked against us, as we reach our later years.

The book's primary goal is to stimulate mental activity, on the part of the elderly relative concerned. This is mental activity triggered from thoughts about the distant past, and thoughts relating to more recent times or the present day.

A secondary goal of *Thinkwich* is to lift the spirits of an elderly relative. By allowing him or her to recall and share with the family, life events from the distant past while enjoying a relatively light mental workout on more general, logic- or memory-related questions.

Without further definitive study, it is impossible to say for sure whether a family's use of this book and the techniques it incorporates, would contribute to a senior's level of mental acuity and cognition. Until such studies are carried out, we must assume though, based on our own research that every little helps.

Maintaining a Cognitively Stimulating Lifestyle

Much has been written on the importance of trying to lead a cognitively stimulating lifestyle; in the knowledge that the more active we keep our brains, the longer they will last into old age. Taking steps to actively stimulate the brain, is likely to prolong its general usefulness with respect to social interaction and the needs surrounding everyday life.

Depending on the circumstances, such activity may provide an elderly relative with a greater sense of well-being and control over their daily lives.

Maintaining or creating this stimulation for the brain with regard to an aging relative, must in part be driven by the family, of course. This may entail providing a range of crosswords, puzzles, and quizzes, for instance, or simply trying to ensure there is a good deal of regular, engaging contact with the family.

So *Thinkwich* can be seen as having a foot in each camp, as it were, in that it is a *resource* that makes it easier for the family to share *engaging contact* with the senior concerned as and when desired.

[Note: Despite the focus here on cognitive health, it should be remembered that cognitive health, is only one element of overall brain health and well-being]

3. Using *Thinkwich*.

Whether face-to-face, or on a video call with the elderly relative concerned, once you have introduced the idea of *Thinkwich* and hopefully have consent to go ahead, just begin at **TW 1** and start to ask the questions listed. Offering encouragement and praise where you can of course. To avoid fatigue, we recommend covering no more than one question list per session.

In terms of how often to use *Thinkwich*, that's of course ultimately up to you, however the aim should not be to rush through the book at speed. We would suggest based on our experience that once every two or even three weeks is probably best; unless of course the elderly relative concerned requests otherwise.

The book is best used as a *base* around which to build engagement and interaction. In this regard, sharing your own answers to some of the questions can also help, as can asking your own follow-up questions at any point.

It is important to mention also that many of the hints and answers provided are simply *examples* of correct answers; it may be that the senior concerned gives alternative answers to those shown.

Introducing *Thinkwich* to an Elderly Relative

So, how should *Thinkwich* be introduced to an elderly relative? Obviously, this is entirely up to *you*. However, one approach could be to explain, for instance, that you picked up a book of short quizzes with questions about the past and present that might be fun to try out?

The senior should know that the questions are not likely to be overly difficult and also come with hints if needed. Additionally, they should know that *out of respect for privacy, personal questions do not refer to partners.*

4. The Questions.

H = Hint / A = Answer)

CAUTION: *questions below and throughout the book that do not directly involve reminiscence should be avoided in cases of dementia in any of its forms.*

TW1

Try to memorize this card sequence

(You'll be asked again at the end of the quiz!):

7 Hearts, 4 Hearts, 7 Diamonds (repeat x2)

Can you recall a comedy show you used to watch way back when?
If so, can you remember the names of any of the stars involved?

If water is 5..and tea is 3 what is coffee?
H: Letters/Number of letters / A: 6

In which town or city were you born?
Where did you move to next?

In the well-known song, in which US state were the Blue Ridge Mountains?
H: State beginning with V / A: Virginia

Do you recall the names of any vacation or holiday destinations you visited when you were younger?
If so, was any one of these better than the others?

If you take half of a number, add 6 you get 11, what was the number?
H: Same as 11-6 x2 /A:10

Can you remember owning records when you were younger?
If so, can you name any of the groups or singers?

What two colors are most commonly associated with relaxation?
H: b.. / g.. / A: blue / green

Growing up, did your family have a dog or cat? If so, can you remember any names?

Can you think of countries with a total of five letters in their names?

Eg.
H: J.. / E.. / S..
A: Japan/ Egypt/ Spain
Have you been to any of the countries you named?
If so, when?

Can you recall the card sequence from earlier?

TW 2

<u>Try to memorize this safe code:</u>

10 left, 1 right, 10 left (repeat x2)

When you were young, did you have a Saturday job or similar?
If so, can you remember how much it paid?

Can you think of any Latin American dance styles?
Eg.
H: rum.. / sal.. / tan..
A: rumba/ salsa/ tango
Did you ever dance any of these?

Did you ever have an accident in the kitchen?
H: Cut a finger, slipped or dropped something for instance

In which century was the year 1900?
H: Not the eighteenth
A: Nineteenth (Twentieth century began in 1901)

Who was one of Bing Crosby's most famous male co-stars?
H: Fred A.
A: Fred Astaire
Which of the two was known as the better dancer?
H: Most letters in surname / A: Fred Astaire

A very famous female Italian movie star from 1950s with the initials "GL"?
H: Gina Loll.. /A: Gina Lollobrigida
Do you recall any of the movies in which she starred?
H: Notre Dame / A: The Hunchback of Notre Dame
H: Trap_ _ _ /A: Trapeze
Did you see any of her movies?

What hobbies did you have when you were younger?

Can you name any types of pasta?
H: pen.. / sp../ tag..
A: penne /spaghetti/ tagliatelle

Do you remember ever hiking or climbing a big mountain?
If so, where was it?
Where were you living at that time?

Can you recall the code to the safe from earlier?

TW 3

Try to memorize this safe code:

4 right, 2 right, 2 left (repeat x2)

Can you recall the star signs of anyone in your family?

What two numbers are used in the Binary number system?
H: One and ….
A: Ones and zeroes.

When you were young did you have a dream of what you wanted to be when you grew up?

In which industry does the binary number system play a very important part?
H: Com../ A: Computing

Do you remember the names of any of your P.E (physical education) teachers from school?
Was there a P.E activity you liked best?

How many star signs can you name?
Eg.
H: Pi.. / Aq.. / Le.
A: Pisces/ Aquarius/ Leo

When you were younger, were you were aware of any important world events and if so, did you watch them on TV?

Eg. The Coronation of Elizabeth II for instance.

How many days in seven weeks?
H: 7 x 7
A: 49

Can you remember ever going sledding?
If so where did you go to do this?

Can you name any of the USA's New England colonies?
Eg.
H: Con.. /Mass../Rho..
A: Connecticut/ Massachusetts/ Rhode Island

Can you recall the code to the safe from earlier?

TW 4

<u>Try to memorize this safe code:</u>

9 right, 9 left, 1 left (repeat x2).

Do you remember any well-known authors from when you were younger?
Did you read any of their books?
Are you reading or listening to a book at the moment?
If so what is it about?

Which of these is odd one out and why?
wash/ catch/ rinse/spin
H: Three are part of a household chore
A: catch. Not part of a washing cycle.
Did you ever do or help do the washing?

Can you picture a local store where you used to buy candy when you were younger?
If so, where was it located?

If you juggle tomatoes on Tuesdays and watches on Wednesday- what might you juggle on Fridays?
H: Something with 'f' as the first letter.
Eg. A: fish

When you were young did you have a favorite breakfast cereal?

Can you recall some of the popular breakfast cereals from that time?
What did you usually drink at family dinner time?

Can you name any social media platforms?
H: Face.. /Tw../ Insta..
A: Facebook / Twitter / Instagram
Are you a user of any social media platforms?

Do you remember the color of your childhood bedroom?
Can you recall the position of the window and the bed from the doorway?

Can you give two examples of the use of the word 'key'?
H: door/ map
A: key to a door/ information inset on a map

Have you ever played chess, or bridge ?
If so, where did you play?
What other board or card games did you play?

Can you recall the code to the safe from earlier?

TW 5

Try to memorize the dimensions of this triangle:

3 x 2 x 6 (repeat x2)

Albert was the first name of a famous physicist, what was his surname?
H: Ein.. / A: Einstein
Do you know his country of birth?
H: G.. /A: Germany

Can you remember the names of any brands of ice cream you used to eat when you were younger?

What is *rising* as a result of the icecaps melting due to global warming?
 H: s.. l.. / A: sea levels

Can you remember singing or acting in any plays or shows at school or elsewhere?

Another word for brothers or sisters? H: sib..
A: siblings

Did you learn any languages at school?
If so, can you name any words in that language and their meaning in English?

Can you think of any words that have a similar sounding ending to 'ouch' ?
Eg.
H: cou../ vou../ lou.. /   A: couch/ vouch/ louch

Do you remember the name of someone you liked at school.. or that liked you ?
If so where was the school?
Approximately how old were you?

Can you name any countries in South America?
Eg.
H: Per.. / Bol.. / Bra.. A: Peru/ Bolivia/ Brazil

What is one of the most famous tourist attractions in Peru?
Eg.
H: Machu P.. A: Machu Picchu

When you were young, did you ever go swimming at a public swimming pool?
If so, where was that?

Can you recall the dimensions of the triangle from earlier?

TW 6

<u>Try to memorize the dimensions of this box:</u>

4 x 3 x 1 (repeat x2).

Do you remember where you were/ what you were doing when JF Kennedy was shot?

Architecturally, which offers the greatest strength: a square, a triangle or a circle?
H: Less than four sides.
A: triangle.

Do you know the sum of all angles in any triangle?
H: Highest score on a dart board too!
A: 180 degrees

When you were young did you have a paddling pool or swimming pool?
If so where were you living at the time?
Do you recall who else used to swim or play in the pool with you?

What was the nickname given to the process of the UK leaving the EU?
H: Br../ A: Brexit
Can you remember the year in which it happened?
H: Not 2019! A: 2020

Do you remember what you used to do in the evenings before TV came along?
Do you remember when your family got its first TV?

Yuri was this famous person's first name.. so what was his surname?
H: Gag.. / A: Gagarin
Why was he famous?
H: First person to do this special thing.
A: First person travel to outer space.

Did you often host dinner parties for your friends?
Can you name a few of these friends?

Can you finish the name of either of these famous bands?:
Rolling / Fleetwood
H: Rolling St.. / Fleetwood Ma..
A: Rolling Stones / Fleetwood Mac
Do you remember listening to music from these groups?
Can you remember the names of any of the songs?

Can you remember ever waiting for a school bus?
Where was that?
If not, how did you get to school?

Can you recall the dimensions of the box from earlier?

TW 7

Try to memorize these recipe ingredients:

3 eggs, 1 cup milk, 1 tablespoon butter (repeat x2).

Which did you like best at school—math or English?
Do you remember the teacher's name?

Can you name any member of the Rolling Stones?
Eg. H: Mick J.. A: Mick Jagger

What was a mangle used for?
H: Manually doing something that is now very easy by machine.
A: Wringing water out of wet clothes.
Did your family have a mangle when you were younger?
Why were they dangerous to use?

What do the letters LP stand for in terms of vinyl records?
H: long p.. / A: long play
Did you have a big record collection?
Can you remember any of the records you owned?

Do you remember the name of any perfume or aftershave you used when you were younger?

Add the number of months in a year, to the number of days in a week and add 2. What number do you get? A:21

As a child, can you remember visiting a library?
Where was that?

Do you know the name of the worlds' longest river?
H: N.. / A: Nile.
Can you guess roughly how long is it?
A: Around 6500 km/ 4000 Miles.

Do you remember playing any games in the school playground?
What games did you play?
Do you remember any friends you used to play with at school?

Can you name any of Canada's provinces?
H: Alb../ British C.../ Ont..
A: Alberta / British Columbia/ Ontario

Can you recall the recipe ingredients from earlier?

TW 8

Try to memorize this task list:

Check mail, water plants, change sheets (repeat x2)

Can you complete this phrase?: "Practice makes ..."
H: per.. A: perfect

Did you like to dance?
If so, what were some of the styles you liked and where did you to go to dance?

What speed did LP records used to spin at? Was it approximately 33 or 45 revolutions per minute?
H: Slowest spinning A: 33 RPM.
How big in inches were these records?   A: 12 inches.

Can you name some past or present foreign leaders?
Which countries do or did they represent?
Eg.
H: Emmanuel M.. , F..
A: Emmanuel Macron, France.

How many Beatles songs can you remember?
Eg. H: Let .. / Hey ... / Yellow ...
A: Let It Be/ Hey Jude/ Yellow Submarine.

Which is the largest country in the world?
H: R.. A: Russia
Which do you think are the next two largest countries?
H: Ca../ Ch.. /A: Canada/ China.

Can you remember the names of any classmates from your earliest school days?

Does the Moon go around the Earth or the other way around?
H: The smaller of the two goes around the other.
A: The Moon goes around the Earth.
Approximately how many days does it take?
H: 17 or 27? / A: 27

Can you remember the names of some of your aunts and uncles?
What about any nephews or nieces?

Can you recall the task list from earlier?

TW 9

Try to memorize these trip details:

Spain on 1st, Germany on 2nd, Italy on 3rd

In the song by Bill Haley and the Comets.. what did they "rock around"?
H: The cl.. / A: The clock.

On a clock face what number is directly opposite 2?
A: 8.

Did you have any favorite books when you were younger?

Can you complete these lyrics from a famous song:
" Starry ….. night "
H: st.. / A: starry
What was the name of the song itself ?
H: Vin.. / A: Vincent

Do you remember saving money in a piggy bank or money box?
If so, can you remember what colour it was?
Did you save a lot of money?

Can you complete this: "Snow White and the …"
H: 7 of something/ dwar... A: seven dwarves).

Can you remember back to the first time you learned to ride a bicycle?
Did you manage by yourself or did someone help you?

Can you finish this line from one of Shakespeare's plays: "To be or not to be..."
H: "That is the.." / A: "That is the question."
Do you remember the name of the play concerned?
H: Ham.../A: Hamlet

Do you remember climbing trees, or playing in a garden when you were younger?
Where was that?

What is the name of the main gas taken in by plants?
H: Carbon D .. A: Carbon Dioxide.
Do you know the short name for Carbon Dioxide?
H: C _ 2 A: CO 2

Can you recall the trip details from earlier?

TW 10

<u>Try to memorize these trip details:</u>

Hotel 3 nights, log cabin 3 nights,
cruise home. (repeat x2)

Do you remember the last time you voted?
Where were you?
Can you recall who was in power?

Which has higher numbers Fahrenheit or Centigrade?
H: Add 451 to get the name of a novel.
A: Fahrenheit.
Do you know who wrote the novel Fahrenheit 451?
H: Ray B .. / A: Ray Bradbury

What is likely to be the next number?
2   5   8   11 _
H: Add 3 / A: 14

Did you ever fly in a plane that had propellers?
If so, do you remember where you were going?

Who is the first president or prime minister you can
remember being in charge of your Country?

Do you remember any really bad weather events that
affected your local area in the past?

Can you finish this letter sequence? Y M _ _
(it is also a popular song from a while back)
A: C A
Do you know what those letters stand for?
H: Young Men's …
A: Young Men's Christian Association.

Who has more ribs.. men, women or is it the same?
A: Despite the stories, its the same!

When you were young, were you more afraid of spiders,
the dark or neither?

What city in northern England was the home town of
unquestionably the most successful band of all time?
H: L.. / A: Liverpool
What was the band's name?
H: The Be.../ A: The Beatles
Did you ever watch the Beatles live? Or on TV?

Can you recall the trip details from earlier?

TW 11

Try to memorize this sequence of letters:

A Z B   (repeat x2).

Can you remember any famous people from way back with the first name 'John'?
Eg.
H: US president in the 1960s? / A: John F Kennedy
H: Actor appearing in many westerns- surname beginning with 'W'.?
A: John Wayne.

Try to picture yourself looking at the front of a house you lived in as a child. Where was the house?
Was it made of brick, stone or wood?
Can you remember any friends who lived close by?

If red is 4, blue is 5 what is purple likely to be?
H: Number of letters in word +1
A: 7.

Can you remember eating school dinners?
Was there something on the menu that you really hated having to eat?

Which is fastest, the speed of light or the speed of sound?
H: In a thunderstorm, which comes first, the sound of
thunder or the flash of lightning?
A: The speed of light is fastest.
Do you know what the speed of light is?
A: 186,000 miles per second.

Did you use to collect things when you were younger?
If so, what did you collect?
How big was your collection?

According to the creation myth where did Adam and Eve
first meet?
H: G.. of E..
A: Garden of Eden

Did you ever have to wear a school tie?
If so do you recall what color it was?

Can you remember the sequence of letters from earlier?

TW 12

Try to memorize this sequence of letters:

C B A (repeat x2).

Do you remember the popular Swedish group from the 1970s and 80s?

H: A... / A: Abba
Can you remember any of Abba's hits?
Eg.
H: Money ... ... / Water..
A: Money money money/ Waterloo

When you were younger, how often did you meet your aunts or uncles?
Do you recall where any of them lived?

What contains calories?
H: F.. & D..
A: Food and drink

What does the phrase 'wet behind the ears mean'
H: Relates to the experience of a person.
A: A person lacking in experience.

Do you ever remember visiting a 'pick-your-own' fruit or vegetable farm?
If so, what was the fruit or vegetable?

How many cartoon characters can you name?
Which of these did you often watch when you were
younger?

How many pounds in a kilogramme?
H: More than 2 but less than 3. /A: 2.2

Did you belong to any clubs, associations or societies
when you were younger?
This could include sports clubs too for example?

Which port did the Titanic sail from on maiden its voyage?
H: Long word beginning with 'S' / A: Southampton
What was its intended destination?
H: New … / A: New York.

Can you put names to these initials of two famous jazz
artists from way back? "LA" " EF"
H: Louis A.. /Ella F..
A: Louis Armstrong / Ella Fitzgerald

Can you remember the sequence of letters from earlier?

TW 13

Try to memorize this code:

1A 2B 26Z (repeat x2)

Can you remember the names of any of the clothing stores you shopped at when you were younger?
If so, in which town or city were they?

What communication device immediately preceded the telephone?
H: Also begins with T / A: telegraph.

As a child, were there any foods you didn't like?

How many US presidents can you remember?
Eg.
H: JF.. / Ob....
A: JF Kennedy, Obama.

What was your first job after leaving school?

Which word is most likely next in this sequence:
up/down, in/out, top/....?
H: Begins with 'b' /A: bottom

What kind of music did you like when you were in your teens?

What is the 10th letter of the alphabet? A: J

When you were young do you remember getting pocket money or an allowance?
If so, did you have to earn it?
Do you remember how much it was?

Can you multiply 18 x 3 in your head?
H: 17 x 3 = 51
A: 54

Can you name any cities in northern England?
H: Liv../ She.. / Lee..
A: Liverpool / Sheffield / Leeds

Can you remember the code from earlier?

TW 14

Try to memorize this code:

020304 (repeat x2)

What comes next in this phrase?: "Sticks and stones ….
… .. "
H: may break … … /A: "may break my bones, but names
will never hurt me".
Can you explain in your own words what it means?
H: It's related to other people calling us names.
A: If someone calls us a bad name it won't hurt us
physically.

Did you ever ride on a motorbike? If so where were you at
the time?

Can you name any deserts?
Eg.
H: Sa.... / Go .. A: Sahara / Gobi
Do you know which is the World's biggest desert?
H: Ant.. / A: Antarctic Desert

Who was your first real best friend?
What kind of things did you often do together?

Can you name any famous composers?
H: Moz.. /A: Mozart
H: Andrew L. W
A: Andrew Lloyd Webber.

Have you ever been to any big sporting events?
If so, when was that?

What is the main drug in coffee?
H: Caf..
A: Caffeine.
What is one of the side effects of Caffeine?

In the past, did you follow certain fashion trends?
Eg.
Mini-skirts, bell bottoms, platform heels, for instance.
If so, which?

Did you or do you often drink coffee or tea?
If so which brands do you like?

Can you name any five, five letter words?

Can you remember the code from earlier?

TW 15

<u>Try to memorize this sequence of playing cards:</u>

10 Hearts, 9 Diamonds, 8 Spades (repeat x2)

Can you remember the names of any of your bosses, from jobs you had in the past?

What is the number likely to follow in this sequence?
2   6   18   _   / H: x3 / A: 54

Which newspapers did you use to read ?
Did you get them delivered? If not, where did you go to buy them?

Is ice less dense than water?
A: Yes
What is one main reason that we know this?
A: Ice floats (eg. Icebergs).

Can you remember the name of your first bank?
Where was the branch in question?

Complete these:
"Come rain or .. " /   " fish & .. "
H: come s..   / A: come shine / H: c.. / A: chips
Can you remember the taste of fish and chips?
If so where did you use to buy them?

Can you recall a very famous mythical London detective?
H: SH /A: Sherlock Holmes
On which London street did he live?
H: A person who makes bread. / A: Baker Street.

Can you recall the now famous phrase Holmes often used
when talking to his sidekick Watson?
H: "It's elementary … "
A: "It's elementary my dear Watson"

Would you say you have 'Green Fingers'?
Either way, did you use to keep house plants or have a
garden?
Where was that?

Can you recall the card sequence from earlier?

TW 16

Try to memorize this sequence of playing cards:

9 Clubs, 9 Spades, 8 Hearts (repeat x2).

When you were young, did you use to read comics?
If so which ones?

Can you complete this phrase?
"All's well ..."
H: That ends ....
A: That ends well.

Can you remember the model of the first car you owned?
If so, what colour was it?

Can you name any famous tennis players?
Eg.
H: Roger ... / Venus ....
A: Roger Federer / Venus Williams.

Did you ever meet or know personally, anyone famous or at least famous in your local area?

Can you name any countries beginning with P?
Eg.
H: Pol... / Port.../ A: Poland / Portugal.

Did you have any special skills when you were younger? (Dressmaking, cooking, sewing, car mechanics or home DIY for instance).

Can you explain the difference between diameter and radius?

H: This relates to certain ways to measure the size of a circle.

A: Diameter is the distance across a circle, radius is distance to the center of a circle.

Have you ever played any musical instruments? If so where did you play?

Do you remember using a skipping/ jump rope or firing a catapult?

Can you recall the card sequence from earlier?

TW 17

Try to memorize this sequence of playing cards:

5 Diamonds, 4 Hearts, 3 Spades (repeat x2).

Did you listen to any radio programs when you were younger? If so what were they about?

If it takes three eggs and half a cup of milk to make one omelette.. what would it take to make four omelettes?
A: Twelve eggs/ two cups of milk.

Can you remember any famous sports personalities from your youth?

Do you remember using any local takeout food outlets when you were younger?
Where were you living at the time?

Can you name the biggest American movie awards show?
H: The Os...
A: The Oscars.
Did you ever watch this award show on TV?

Which do you prefer hot or cold weather?
Where is the coldest, or hottest place you have ever been?

When you were younger did you ever sleep in a tent?
Where was that?

Can you remember where you were during the televised
moon landing in the 1960s?
Did you watch the event?

One of the most famous comic actors ever to appear in
silent movies?
H: CC / A: Charlie Chaplin

Can you name other stars from the silent movies era?
H: Greta G. / Douglas F. / Buster K.
A: Greta Garbo/ Douglas Fairbanks / Buster Keaton

Can you recall the card sequence from earlier?

TW 18

<u>Try to memorize this task list:</u>

Do washing, cook lunch, tidy house (repeat x2)

Did you ever watch a musical in person or on TV?
Can you name any musicals?
Eg.
H: The Sound ... . / A: The Sound of Music.
H: The Wiz...... .... /A: The Wizard of OZ.

At school do you remember ever being told off by the teacher?
If so what did you do wrong? *If not what was your secret?!*

Can you describe the meaning of the word: 'genesis'?
H: The ori.... of something / A: The origin of something

Do you remember ever going to a zoo? If so, can you recall where it was?

What is most likely to be the missing number?: 5 12 19 _
H: Add seven A: Twenty-six

Did you ever do any charity work or take part in sponsored events for a charity?

What is a word that could be used as a close opposite to 'proud'?

Eg.

H: hum.../ A: humble

H: ash... A: ashamed

Where did your father work?

What was his position?

Can you think of at least two meanings of the word 'move'?

H: Relates to a feeling / A: To feel moved by someone or something.

H: Relates to location /A: Move something to a different place.

Can you recall the task list from earlier?

TW 19

Try to memorize this sequence of playing cards:
3 Spades, 4 Clubs, 5 Clubs (repeat x2).

Can you picture any rivers or streams you used to play in or walk along when you were younger?
If so, where were they?

If a clock shows 3.15pm what time will it be in in 63 minutes?
H: How many minutes in an hour? then add 3
A: 4.18pm.

Which season do you like best and why?

Do you know what a prime number is?
H: It can only be divided by …
A: A number divisible only by 1 and itself.

At school, which subjects were you best at?
Do you remember who taught you in the classes concerned?

What are most likely the next two letters
in this sequence: A C E _ _
H: Just skip next letter / A: G and I

What was the last sport you played?
Where did you play it?

Which numbers are Prime numbers odd numbers or even numbers?
H: Can only be divided by the number itself and 1.
A: Odd numbers

Can you remember any lines from well-known poems, plays or movies?
Eg.
H: "Now is the winter of … ...."
A: "Now is the winter of our discontent"
(Shakespeare: Richard III)
H: "Here's looking … … …"
A: "Here's looking at you kid" (Casablanca)
Who said *that* famous line by the way?
H: Humphrey B. A: Humphrey Bogart

Can you recall the card sequence from earlier?

TW 20

Try to memorize the dimensions of this box:

10 x 5 x 6 (repeat x2).

Were you ever in the armed services?
If so what was your rank and what did you do?
Where were you based?

Which everyday household item is often associated with a witch?
H: Used to sweep the floor.
A: broom.

Do you remember how many times it took you to pass your driving test?
If you didn't take a driving test, how did you usually get around?

What is one way to find the age of a tree?
A: Cut it down and count the rings.

Roughly how long in miles is a marathon race?
H: 22, 24, 26 ? / A: 26 miles.
Did you ever run or watch a marathon race?

Do you have a favorite TV programme?
If so, how often do you watch it?

Can you name any voice activated AI digital assistance devices?

H: Ale_ / Si_ _ / A: Alexa/ Siri

Do you regularly use one of these, or another?

What kind of thing do you ask the AI assistant about?

Do you remember visiting your grandparents house?

Where did they live?

Which is likely to be the missing number? :

10 17 24 .. 38

Are you aware of the early occupations of any of your grandparents?

Can you recall the dimensions of the box from earlier?

TW 21

<u>Try to memorize this group of animals:</u>

Tiger, Lion, Horse (repeat x2).

Do you remember ever attending a school sports day?
whether at your own school, or for someone else.
Can you recall the name of the school and where it was?

Can you explain the word 'fraction'?
A: A part of something

Do you remember making packed lunches for school?
Or helping children with homework?

What is the main job of a cobbler?
H: repairing ....
A: repairing shoes.

Can you picture attending any birthday parties when you
were younger?
If so, do you remember whose party it was?

Can you name any well-known political activists or civil
rights leaders?
Eg.
H: ML _ / Malcolm _ / Emmeline P
A: Martin Luther King /Malcolm X/ Emmeline Pankhurst.

Can you remember the brand names of any shampoo or other hair products you used in the past?

How many states are there in the USA ?
H: More than 48 less than 52? /A: 50

Can you name any of Shakespeare's plays?
Eg.
H: Ham..../ King … / Romeo ….
A: Hamlet/ King Lear/ Romeo & Juliet.
Did you ever watch any of them?

In medicine what do the letters GP stand for?
H: general …………..
A: general practitioner.
How many letters in the word 'practitioner'?
H: More than 10!
A: 12

Can you remember the animals from earlier?

TW 22

Try to memorize this group of animals:

koala, kangaroo, wolf (repeat x2)

How did you get to your primary or elementary school?
Where was the school?

Can you name any of the different varieties of apple?
Eg.
H: Granny …. / Golden …. /Bald ….
A: Granny Smith/ Golden Delicious/ Baldwin

What was the most dangerous thing you ever did?
Eg.
H: Parachute jump, skiing, driving for instance.

Can you name any famous painters?
Eg.
H: Pic... / Mon.. / John ….
A: Picasso /Monet/ John Constable

Can you think of a really great movie you have seen in the past?
Was that on TV or at the cinema?

In which sport can you score a birdie, or an eagle?
H: Use a club to hit the ball / A: golf
In golf, which is the best a birdie or eagle?
H: Golden ... /A : eagle

Do you remember being taught handwriting or art at school?
If so, do you recall any of the teacher's names?

Who was the other half of this comedy duo: Laurel and..?
H: H.. / A: Hardy
Which one of the two was the thinnest?
H: L.. / A: Laurel

Can you give the name of two places you have lived in?
Which was earliest?
Which did you like best?

Can you remember the animals from earlier?

TW 23

Try to memorize these strange vegetables:

Green potato, blue onion, red celery (repeat x2)

Did you ever play the Lottery? or Bingo?
If so did you have any success?
Where were you at the time?

The White House broke with tradition in 2022 by flying its flags at half-mast; why was this?
H: QE / A: In memory of Queen Elizabeth II.

Can you remember any children's nursery rhymes?
Eg.
H: Old Mc / A: Old Mc Donald had a farm.
H: Twinkle / A: Twinkle twinkle little star.

If A = 1 and B = 2 what number would you most likely associate with the letter X?
H: Z would be 26.
A: 24.

Did you or someone in a car you were traveling in ever get stopped by the Police?
Can you remember why and where you were at the time?

Where would you expect to see Mr Spock?
H: American TV series set in space.
A: Star Trek.
What was special about Spock's appearance?
H: pointed .. / pointed ears.

Did your mother or father play sports?
If so, which sports and at what level?

Can you think of two more words to continue this series:
car, boat, train, bus.. ?
Eg.
H: flies/ goes underwater.
A: airplane / submarine.

Can you remember any heroes or heroines from the books
you read when you young?

Can you remember the strange vegetables from earlier?

TW 24

<u>Try to memorize the details of this scheduled meeting</u>:

John Smith 3rd floor, 2pm. (repeat x2)

Did you ever go fishing, skiing, climbing or diving?
If so where was that?

Can you name any four capital cities?
Eg.
H: Wa /Lon
A: Washington DC / London

Do you remember the names of any doctors you were registered with in the past?

What is likely next in this sequence?
A D G _ ?
H: Skip two letters
A: J.

Do you have early memories of going to church?
If so, where was that?

Kermit the frog belonged to which group of characters?
H: The M...
Did you ever watch the Muppet show?

How many words can you think of that can describe a person's appearance?
Eg.
H: pr.. / attr../ ug.. / A: pretty, attractive, ugly etc.

Where were you born?
Which was the closest major city?

Can you name any famous horse races?
Eg.
H: Melbourne ... /A: Melbourne Cup
H: Kentucky .. /A: Kentucky Derby
H: The Grand … / A: The Grand National
Did you ever go to watch a horse race?

Were you ever stung by a bee or a wasp, or bitten by a dog or cat?
If so where were you at the time?

Can you remember the meeting details from earlier?

TW 25

<u>Try to memorize this sequence of events and the timing:</u>

Car accident 10.00 am, police called 10.05 am,

police arrive 10.15 am. (repeat x2)

Can you name any places beginning with the letter 'B'?
Eg.
H: Birm./ Berm../ Belg..
A: Birmingham/Bermuda /Belgium.

What was the name of your first boyfriend of girlfriend?
Where did you first meet him or her?

Did you ever chop logs, cut down a tree or cut someone's hair ?
Where were you at the time ?

Can you think of words that describe someone's character ?
Eg.
H: rel../ gen.. / loy..
A: reliable/ generous/ loyal.
How might a friend describe your character do you think?

When you were young did you or a friend have a tree house?
Where were you living at the time?

A famous Australian female singer: Kylie ...
H: Mino .. /A: Kylie Minogue.
She also starred in which Australian soap opera?
H: Neig.. / A: Neighbours.

Were you on any sports teams in high-school or college?
If so do you remember some of the best matches you
played?
Did your team win?

What does the F stand for in F1?
H: form... / A: formula
Which location is considered to be the host of the most
popular F1 race? H: Mon... /A: Monaco.

Did you ever go to the ballet or a concert?
If so where and when was that?

Can you name any of the most famous US baseball
players?
H: Babe ... / Ted W... / Barry ...
A: Babe Ruth / Ted Williams / Barry Bonds
Did you ever watch a baseball game live?
Where was that?

Can you recall the events and timing from earlier?

TW 26

<u>Try to memorize this computer password:</u>

147*741 (repeat x2)

Did you ever jump on a trampoline?
If so, can you remember where you were at the time?

Can you name any famous F1 drivers?
H: Michael S.. / Ayrton S.. / James H.. / Mario A..
A: Michael Schumacher/ Ayrton Senna/ James Hunt/
Mario Andretti.

Did you ever sing in public or at school?
What were you singing?

The name of the most famous Paris art gallery?
H: The L..
A: The Louvre
Can you name a movie in which it featured?
Eg.
H: The Da ..
A: The Da Vinci Code

Do you know the French word for love?
A: l'amour
Do you know any other French words?

Have you ever given a wedding speech or spoken publicly in another setting?

Who was the famous singer known as 'old blue eyes'?
H: Frank ..
A: Frank Sinatra
Can you remember any of his songs?
Eg.
H: My .. /New .. /Fly ..
A: My Way/ New York, New York/Fly Me To The Moon.

As far as you can remember, have you ever had stitches or worn a plaster cast?
If so why, what happened?

Can you remember the computer password from earlier?

TW 27

<u>Try to memorize this computer password:</u>

8899* (repeat x2)

Are you left or right-handed?
Do you know approximately what percentage of people are left-handed?
H: Under 20%! / A: 10 %.

How many different musical genres can you name?
Eg.
H: R.. / P.. / J.. / A: Rock /Pop/ Jazz..

What are some of the countries you have travelled to?
Can you remember any famous places you visited whilst you were there?

Can you name any English premier league UK football teams?
Eg.
H: West.. / Liv.. / Ch.. / A: West Ham /Liverpool /Chelsea
Did you ever watch a live football/ soccer match?
If so where was that?

Have you ever been on cruise or a safari?
If so, where did you go?

In the well-known song, where did the "Raindrops keep falling on ..."?
H: m _ _ _ _ _
A: "my head".
Do you know who the original singer was?
H: B.J ... / A: B.J Thomas.

Do remember the name of your music teacher at school?

What is Melanin?
H: Substance in the body that produces something.
A: Melanin produces hair, skin and eye pigmentation.

Can you remember the computer password from earlier?

TW 28

Try to memorize this computer password:

200+002

Have you ever been roller skating or ice skating?
If so, do you remember where?

Who was the first man on the moon?
H: Neil … / A: Neil Armstrong.
What was the number of the Apollo rocket used? A: 11.
Do you remember the year? A: 1969

Ever used a canoe, sailed a boat or driven a truck?
If so, where were you at the time?

What is most likely to be the next number in this sequence:
3   7   15 _ ?
H: Double + _ ? A: 31

Can you name some of the most well known NFL football
teams in the USA?
H: Dallas C... / New England P...
A: Dallas Cowboys / New England Patriots
Can you name some past or present NFL players?
H:. Bart S…/ Tom B… / Jerry R.. /
A: Bart Starr/ Tom Brady/ Jerry Rice.

Have you ever made a flower arrangement, or dug a
vegetable garden?
If so, where were you living at the time?

In which decade was the Watergate scandal?
H: Not 1960's / A: 1970s
Which newspaper published the story concerned?
H: WP
A: Washington Post
Who was the US president at the time?
H: RN /A: Richard Nixon

Did you keep a journal or diary when you were younger?
If so, how often did you write in it?

Who directed the movie 'Psycho'?
H: AH
A: Alfred Hitchcock
Did you watch any Hitchcock movies, if so which ones?

Can you remember the computer password from earlier?

TW 29

<u>Try to memorize these race results:</u>

Driver one: 51 minutes, Driver two: 52 minutes,

Driver three: <u>63</u> minutes (repeat x2)

Have you ever darned socks, mended clothes
or caught a fish?
If so, where were you at the time?

Which type of cuisine is famous for its tacos and burritos?
H: M ..
A: Mexican

Did you write, or ever want to write a book?
If so, about what?
If not, was there something else that you always wanted to
do?

Can you name any two lakes in Switzerland?
Eg.
H: Lake Gen.. /Lake Zur...
A: Lake Geneva/ Lake Zurich

Can you recall any popular beaches you often visited
when you were younger?
If so where were they?

In which game would you hit something made of feathers?
H: bad... / A: badminton.
Did you ever play badminton, or tennis?
If so, where was that?

What is one of your earliest memories?

Which letter is most likely next in this sequence:
C A N D _
H: Once added it spells a word. / A: Y

Do you remember ever travelling on a ferry?
If so, where were you going from and to?

Can you remember the race results from earlier?

TW 30

<u>Try to memorize this weather forecast:</u>

Monday: mild. Tuesday: typhoon. Wednesday: windy.
(repeat x2)

What is the official name for a barrel maker?
H: Car model, Mini C.. / Boxer, Henry C..
A: Cooper.

Would you find New England on the east or west of the USA?
H: Not as hot there.
A: East.

What is the farthest you have been from your home country?
How long did you stay there?

Can you recall the names of any well-known Glenn Miller tunes?
Eg.
H: " in the .." / A: in the mood
Do you remember any other big band celebrities?
Eg.
H: Benny G.. / A: Benny Goodman

Can you picture a game, toy or doll from your childhood?

Can you name some of the main things people now use their mobile/cell phones for?

Eg.

H: ca.. / ga.. /mov.. /mes...

A: calls /games / movies /messaging.

How do you feel about new technology?

In the past were you good at cooking? If so, what were some of the things you liked to prepare?

Either way, what is one of your all-time favorite things to eat?

Who was Tarzan's girlfriend?

H: J.. / A: Jane

Do you remember the chimpanzee's name?

H: Chee.. / A: Cheetah.

Can you remember who played Tarzan in the black and white movies from way back when?

H: Johnny W...

A: Johnny Weissmuller

Can you remember the weather forecast from earlier?

Finally, if there is one piece of advice you could give to a young person today, what would it be?

Feedback

While *Thinkwich* is a published book, it is still, to a degree, work in progress. With your help, we hope to make it even better. We gratefully welcome any and all general feedback, which will be taken into account in any revisions or new publications.

Objective Data Feedback

We are especially interested in finding out how *you* chose to use the book in terms of an aging relative. This is as specifically, in terms of how often *Thinkwich* was used and whether you noticed any change in mood or level of engagement for instance; or other observations that you considered noteworthy.

This is to help us collate more objective data around the effectiveness of the questioning format incorporated in the book. Any information provided will be treated in the strictest confidence; personal information provided will not be made known to others.

Please use *Thinkwich@gmail.com* to share any thoughts, and again, many thanks.

To be kept up-to-date on further publications of *Thinkwich, please let us know using the same email address.*

<u>Making Connections</u>

As part of our effort to extend the reach of *Thinkwich*, we are looking to make connections with organizations focused on the well-being and support of the elderly. If you represent such an organization, we would be very pleased to hear from you.

Effectiveness Trials?

As previously outlined, *Thinkwich* incorporates a novel questioning format, where questions about the distant past are interleaved with more general, memory- or logic-based questions. It is hoped that one day we may see formal effectiveness trials of this questioning format, confirming its potential value in the fight against early stage cognitive decline.

About the Author

A.C French lives on Jeju Island, off the coast of South Korea. In his late fifties, married and joint custodian of the second love of his life: a Chipin named Minnie.

In place of formal qualifications in the mental health and well-being of the elderly, there is an unending desire to find novel solutions to problems, particularly when those problems are seen to affect those closest to him.

In his free time, he can be found cycling around the Island and also developing disruptive ideas that he believes will make the world a better place.

Contact email address Thinkwich@gmail.com

Information Sources Used

A Neurologist's Tips to Protect Your Memory.
https://www.nytimes.com/2022/07/06/well/mind/memory-loss-prevention.html

What Is Mild Cognitive Impairment?
https://www.nia.nih.gov/health/what-mild-cognitive-impairment

Memory Problems: What is and isn't normal aging.
https://my.clevelandclinic.org/health/articles/11826-memory-problems-what-is-normal-aging-and-what-is-not

Passage of time: why people with dementia switch back to the past.
https://theconversation.com/passage-of-time-why-people-with-dementia-switch-back-to-the-past-45159

How Memories Are Made: Stages of Memory Formation.
https://lesley.edu/article/stages-of-memory

The Effectiveness on Reminiscence Therapy
https://www.frontiersin.org/articles/10.3389/fpsyg.2021.709853/full

What is Reminiscence Therapy?
https://www.verywellmind.com/how-reminiscence-therapy-works-5214451

US Based organization providing information and advice across all areas relating to ageing.
https://acl.gov/about-acl/administration-aging

UK based organisation providing information and advice across all areas relating to ageing.
https://www.ageuk.org.uk/information-advice/health-wellbeing/mind-body/mental-wellbeing/

Canada based organization providing extensive resources and information to those working in support of healthy ageing.
https://healthyagingcore.ca/allied-and-partner-organizations/

Canadian Coalition For Seniors Mental Health
https://ccsmh.ca/

www.ingramcontent.com/pod-product-compliance
Lightning Source LLC
Chambersburg PA
CBHW060438290526
45791CB00002B/984